SAFETY AND HEALTH AFFAIRS FOR SUCCESS

Creating A Safe and Healthy Environment

BY

DR. CHARLES LEO

TABLE OF CONTENT

INTRODUCTION

Safety is the state of being protected from dangers, damage, or harm to life and property. Safety is a very important thing that every right-minded person seeks continually, Safety is everybody's responsibility and should be widely observed by everybody organization. People are expected to keep and carry out safety rules and precautions irrespective of their position, rank and status. For instance:

- The use of seat belt when driving
- Not driving when drunk
- The use of helmet safety boot in the workshop and site even during inspections.
- Keeping to road signs and traffic light sign
- Using the pedestrian bridge where it is provided for
- Switch-off every element appliance before leaving the office
- No fighting
- No running on staircase
- No smoking where it could ignite fire etc.

In safety profession, I have dear it sad that every accident is avoidable. This is a proven fact because if every one of us is cautious and take safety as our responsibility of ensuring that safety rules and regulations in our homes, offices, roads, schools etc. are adequately observed, the rate of accident will drastically be reduced. We shall be concentrating more on the home. This is because it is the starting point, and it involves everyone.

CHAPTER ONE

Home Safety Rules

Many people today feel too comfortable and secure in their homes that they ignore basic safety rules and precautions. Worse still, inexcusable neglect often exists in homes that harbor not only strong and energetic adults, but also children and elderly people who are vulnerable. If we can take steps to learn and adhere to home safety precautions, it will prevent a lot of psychological, material and financial damage. Here are some helpful home safety tips from various experts in homes management.

Home Furnishing Precautions

We must make sure that pieces of furniture are placed in safe position. Furniture should be stable and not wobbly. Shelves should be low enough to avoid the use of a stepstool. Sofas, armchairs, double-sisters dilapidated should be removed or repaired.

Dilapidated and taking roofs

broken windows, doors, damaged floors and falling ceilings should be removed or repaired when noticed before causing accident. All stairs, whether inside or outside the house require stable handrails to prevent a fall off. Ensure that water or oil does not stay on the stairs to prevent slipping and falling.

Electrical Cables and Cords

We must ensure extension cords are hidden to prevent tripping and falling. We must also make sure that furniture is not placed on electrical cords or cable as this way wear them down, resulting in electrical shock. Check cables and cords regularly for any sign of wear and tear. Consult an electrical expert for repair and replacement of any electrical cords and cable. Switch off all electrical appliances before leaving the house. Children are to be cautioned not to play or tamper with electric appliances to avoid damage and electrical shock.

Lighting Precautions

Ensure lighting levels should be fairly consistent throughout the house. People find it difficult to focus when they move from light to dark areas and vice versa. You must keep torchers handy in case of power failure; and often check to ensure batteries are in good condition. Please, avoid candle as much as possible. Make sure there are several night light throughout the house especially near bedroom, bathrooms, staircase and entrances.

Bathroom Precautions

Do not touch any electrical appliances when bathing, keep water heater set to 120. Do not leave a child is learning to bath himself, always remain within arm's reach. Ensure that any medicated soap, detergent, bedroom cleaning supplies and the other harmful substances are carefully stored out of the reach of children. Ensure that safety products, such as grip or grab bars are installed in bathtubs and by the toilet. Bathroom be kept away from water.

Kitchen Precaution

Avoid loose clothing such as night gowns or bathrobes. Regularly clean grease from the stove, oven and exhaust fan, never leave your cooking unattended to. If you must leave the kitchen, lower that heat and take something with you as a reminder pest will go grab it out of curiosity. Also, ensure to keep sharp utensils out of their reach. It is much better to keep young children and pest away from the kitchen entirely. Keep all flammable objects, such window, avoid the use of draperies for such window. Install mini blinds in place of curtains. Curtains may catch fire easily with stove below them. To prevent burns, use clean kitchen safety gloves when taking items in or when removing cooking from the store. Never use gloves soaked with oil or water. While the former gas great potential to catch fire, the latter easily transmit heat. Shield yourself from steam when uncovering food, especially microwave servings. Steam can cause severe burns.

Avoid reaching over the stove for anything while cooking. Keep frequently needed items in other areas of the kitchen. Be careful not to carry a burning pot outside or to the sink. This could escalate the fire. And never attempt to extinguish the oil-fire with water, because the oil will float on the water and the fire get bigger. Keep a lid, baking soda or fire extinguish is made in such a way that it can douse oil-fires.

Hazardous materials

Everyone can attest to that fact that there are several useful materials that can also be hazardous like laundry soaps and detergent, medications, polishes, sprays, kerosene, razor, knife, etc. These are vital substance needed in the homes, but are fatally.

Poisonous when ingested. Little children, especially toddlers and those still crawling tend to put whatever they lay their hands on into their mouths. Thus there's a need to take to those precautions to prevent accidental poisoning.

All hazardous material be kept out of the reach of children. Be careful with house-cleaning chemicals like disinfections and insecticides. Use them as directed by the manufacturers. Allow for sufficient ventilation to minimize toxic fumes. And never attempt to mix different cleaning chemical together. It could lead to deadly chemical reactions. Keep chemical firmly close when you carry them on and recap tightly after each use. Don't leave them on the table or floor even if you are leaving the room for a few minutes. Beware of spraying products especially if they are very appealing to kids but harmful to the eyes and mucous membranes. Try as much as possible to buy products labelled "non-toxic".

CHAPTER TWO

Home Safety Checklist

The Home Safety Council has published a home safety checklist which is to act a guide in keeping our family to buy safety from domestic accidents.

The checklist includes:

1. Have you tested your hot water and turned the temperature of your water heater down to 120For lower to reduce the risk of burns and scalds?
2. Have you had an older phone number (in case of emergency)?
3. Do you have a first aid kit that is easily accessible and stocked with emergency items?
4. Does your family practice a home-fire-escape plan at least twice a year?
5. Are all matches and lighters seared in a locked cabinet?
6. Are dangerous household items such as medicines, toxic bleaches, oven and train clears, and paint solvers, polishes and waxes safety store in a locked cabinet?
7. Do dangerous household and outside products have child-resistance package?
8. Do you keep all plastic wrapping materials, including dry –cleaning bag produce bags and trash bags away from children?
9. Are you careful not to hang pictures or decoration containing ribbon or string on over crib?
10. Have you examined nursery furnishing to be sure they are strong and secure?
11. Have you placed furniture, including ribs and pay pens away from windows to prevent falls?

There may be additional safety needs in your home depending on its age, location, design and add any precautions necessary to make your home accident free.

First Aid

"First aid is a collection of some basic medical items that can be used during emergencies in the home, office or any other accident prone area". Many avoidable fatalities have occurred either due to ignorance of what first aid is or ignorance of the contents and their function. Thus, every parent especially mother must make it an obligation to get a first aid kit in the home and study the uses of each item in it, so as to properly handle emergencies. Here is list of some basic items to including in your first aid kit.

1. First Aid manual
2. Bandage of assorted types for minor cuts and grazes.
3. Triangular bandages for use as slings to support an injured arm or shoulder
4. Elastic wraps-to wrist, ankle, knee and elbow injuries
5. Sterile, non-fluffy, absorbent gauze pads in two and four inch sizes for larger cuts and grazes
6. Adhesive tape to keep gauze in place
7. Scissors to cut tape or clothes
8. Safety pins in variety of sizes to fasten splints and bandages
9. Antiseptic wipes (alcohol free) to disinfect wounds or clean hands
10. Cold packs for icing injuries
11. Tweezes for removing splinters, foreign objects, bee stingers
12. Rubber gloves to protect hand and reduce the risk of infection when treating open wounds.
13. Petroleum jelly
14. Calamine lotion
15. Hydrocortisone cream to relieve irritation from rashes
16. Emergency foil blanket
17. Torch/flashlight

18. Paracetamol and Acetaminophen / Ibuprofen for pain relieve

19. Antihistamine tablets such as Chlorpheniranime e.g. Portion for allergic reactions

20. Antihistamine cream for insect bites (but not for use on broken or infected skin).

CHAPTER THREE

How Do I Get a First Aid Kit?

Well it is advisable you make up a kit yourself, based on your family size need. But in case you don't want to go through the hassles of doing it yourself, some pharmaceutical stores sell ready-made first aid kit all affordable rates. Since there is no official standard for first aid kits, the contents of such kits often vary. You should therefore check to ensure the one you're purchasing contains exactly what you need.

Keep your first aid items in a water proof container, large enough for the content to be well arranged so that items can be quickly found when needed. You that items can use a plastic container or box with a closely fitting lid. Ensure the container is labelled so that it can be easily recognized by anybody that needs it.

Again, it's very important to place the first aid box in a center position to make it accessible during serious or small emergencies. It should not be within the reach of children, but still readily accessible. Wherever you choose to place it, it should be dry and cool and this suggest that the bathroom is no ideal.

Ina summary, knowing how to see the contents of the first aid kit is as important as having it. Hence, it's imperative that all adults, older children and teenagers in the house know where the first aid is, what are in it how to use them. This is why it' suggest you remove any use items as soon as possible. Also check expiry date of items regularly so as to discard and replace expired ones.

Health

It is described as the state of a person's body and mind. It is a vital subject that everyone aspiring to be great and successful must diligently concentrate on. Effort should be made to improve and make it a thing of priority. Someone said," If we only know enough, all disease could be preserved and could be Research has shown that were are two basic things that are likely responsible to our state of health poor or good health condition. They are:

1. What we eat and how we eat them
2. Our habit practice

What Wheat

We must pay close attention to what we eat and how we eat them. This is because our health is directly determined by things we eat. We must prepare our bodies for vitality if we are to be effective in carrying out our day to day activity and responsibilities.

Just as we teach our toddlers not to eat any piece of trash found on the ground, so we learnt from the dietary law of nutritional therapy that we have to eat right in order to live well and be protected from diseases.

Nutritional Therapy

1.   Little or no meat: Research has shown that digestion of animal's protein (with the exception of cultured dietary products such as buttermilk and yoghurt) depletes the body's natural supply of pancreatic enzymes believed to be essential for destroying an invading malignancy. Hence, diet therapist often calls for little or no meat.

2. Whole Natural Food: Because processed foods are notoriously void of many of many essential nutrients and many also have cancer-causing additives, innovative doctors stress the importance of whole natural foods in the diet.

3. Raw fruits and vegetables: Most doctor using nutrition therapy, especially cancer, recommend 80 percent or more of fruit and vegetable in diet. Reason: only in raw food are the maximum amount of enzymes, vitamins are preserved. Due to their nutritional value and cleansing effect, raw vegetable juices play a major role in the degenerative disease therapy

4. High fiber content: Research has revealed a definite connection between colon cancer and other degenerative diseases, and the low fiber diet characteristic of highly processed foods. A high fiber diet results in frequent elimination and better cleansing of toxins from the colon. Whole natural food such as whole gains, raw fruits and raw vegetable all have high fiber content.

CHAPTER FOUR

Preservative Additives

Preservative are chemical added to processed food either to prevent quality deterioration or micro-organism growth. Either way they result in extending the sheaf life.

The concern over preservative focuses mostly around three areas

1. Food needs to be decomposed in digestion. And assimilation of food?
2. Since preservation are inorganic chemicals, are our bodies being "embalmed" by them?
3. Many food additives have been found to cause cancer. Do preservatives encourage cancer? Let's examine some of them.

Sodium Nitrite

Most processed meat including hot dogs, hams, bacon and sausages contain sodium nitrite as preservatives. The meat processing industry uses the ingredient as a color fixer to make food look more attractive and appealing. Yet sodium nitrite is a precursor to some potent cancer-causing chemicals that accelerate the formation and growth of cancer cells through the body. According to Mark Adams, author of the grocery warming manual, "When consumers eat sodium nitrite in popular meat formed in the body where they promote the growth of varies cancers".

Sodium Benzoate

Also known as benzoic acid, sodium benzoates are often used as a natural preservative in liquid drinks (soft drinks, juices etc.) and in processed food such as jams, salad dressing and pickles. According to nutrition experts there's little or no evidence that sodium benzoate, cause any problems in people. But when mixed with ascorbic acid (vitamin c), a chemical reaction occurs and benzene is formed. Unfortunately, benzene is a proven cancer-causing chemical. In an effort to make their drinks more nutritious, many soft drink manufacturers in recent years are adding vitamins c to their drinks and juices, since most of these already contain sodium benzoate, the mixture possess serous health risks.

Propionate

Calcium propionate and sodium propionate are mold inhibitors in bread. Propionates have been shown to cause allergic reactions in the gastro intestinal area and migraine headaches.

Flavorings

Flavorings form the largest category of food additives. They are often added to processed foods. Most of these are synthetic. They are not food and tests are revealing their dangers. Common salt (sodium chloride) the oldest flavoring should be taken sparing because it is not food it. It cannot be digested or assimilated. When taken in excess, it causes harm to the heart and robs the body of calcium.

Many other synthetic flavors and flavor enhancers exist. They are used by food producers because consumers have demanded more flavors to tickle their taste buds. These on analysis are found to be detrimental to health. Colorings, days and artificial sweeteners are to be avoided as much as possible.

The bible in Genesis 1:26-31, reveals to humanity how God our Creator has blessed us and given every herb (plant) hearing seed for our meat-for food so as to have a healthy body. And in scientific finding, food has been discovered to contain curative properties. Food is regarded as a potent medicine; people who eat right will build up healthy and strong bodies. Herein are some food and fruit and what they can do in the body.

1. **Juice:** Juices from guava, carrot, cucumber, beet, tomatoes, apples, pawpaw etc. are rich in vitamins and minerals.
2. **Wheat:** Rich in 16 minerals, iron, phosphorus and calcium including vitamin E.

3. **Avocado:** Good for colitis (an inflammatory bowel disease) and ulcers:
4. **Grape:** A good blood purifier; it is also good for catarrh conditions.
5. **Spinach:** Good for blood supply and helps with eye problem, eases the bowels and provides relief from catarrh.
6. **Apple:** Keeps the cardiovascular system healthy by stabilizing blood sugar and lowering blood cholesterol; people who eat more apples have high resistance to cold and upper respiratory ailments. Apple skins are recommended to help control urinary infections.
7. **Melon:** Lowers the rate of lung cancer, rich in beta-carotene also an effective blood thinner.
8. **Papaya (Pawpaw):** High digestive properties with tonic effect on the stomach.
9. **Onion:** A good medicine; lowers blood cholesterol; thins blood retails clotting in the heart; regulates blood sugar and relieves bronchial congestion.
10. **Corn:** Rich in fiber and vitamin.
11. **Cherry:** An excellent blood builder.
12. **Carrots:** Cut down the chance of contacting cancer of the pancreas; good for the eyes and; eaten to prevent constipation; lowers blood cholesterol.
13. **Eggplant (Garden Egg):** for balancing diet that are heavy in starch and protein
14. **Water Melon:** rich in vitamins.
15. **Tomato:** supplies Beta carotene and lycopene (anti-cancer agent)
16. **Spinach:** good for blood supply and eye problem; eases the bowels and provides relief from catarrh.
17. **Honey:** has some disinfectant properties for wound and sores; recommended for the relief of asthma; soothes sore throats; calms nerves and induces sleep. Don't give a child under one year.
18. **Orange:** protects the arteries from disease; fights arterial plaque and lowers blood cholesterol.

19. PERS: a good intestinal and bowel regulator.

20. **Pop Corn:** good source of intestinal roughage.

21. **Pumpkin:** lowers rate of lungs cancer; rich in Beta-carotene.

22. **Cucumbers:** cooling effect on the body; purifying effect on the bowel; used as a digestive aid.

23. **Lemon/ Lime:** help lowers blood cholesterol.

24. **Lettuce:** Promotes good digestive effect in the intestinal tract.

25. **Mushroom:** Lowers blood cholesterol; thins blood and stimulates the immune system.

26. **Olive:** Said to be good heart disease; thins blood; lowers blood pressure and reduce cholesterol.

27. **Pineapple:** Excellent blood builder; used to aid digestion and tackle catarrh condition. It is good for bone building.

28. **Cabbage:** Rich in vitamin; lowers the risk of cancer of the colon; kills bacterial viruses and prevent ulcers.

29. **Garlic:** Stimulates activity of the digestive organs thereby relieving problems associated with poor digestion; it is also used to emulsify cholesterol and loosen it form the arterial walls.

30. **Soya Bean:** Regulates functions of the colon; said to reduce constipation; prevents bowel problems; used to reduce blood cholesterol; regulates sugar; lowers blood pressure; contains a chemical called lignin's that helps to fight breast and colon cancer.

31. **Yoghurt:** Prevent intestinal infection contains chemicals that prevent ulcers; improves bowel functions; lowers blood cholesterol and strengthens the immune system; rich calcium; good for bone for teeth; scientists have found several cancer fighting properties in yoghurt.

Food combination is very vital to understanding how some food should be mixed for health reason. It has been observed that wrong food combination often results in indigestion of poor digestion in our body system. Here in few tips on food combination:

- Acidic fruits like oranges, grapefruits, pineapples, tomatoes are not to be eaten with carbohydrates. This is because it prevents proper digestion; rather take acid fruit 15 30 minutes before meal.

- Don't eat two concentrated proteins at the same meal like not and meats, Egg and milk, cheese and milk, cheese and egg in order to prevent high cholesterol level.

- Don't eat meals (water melon, musk melon, cantaloupe etc.) with other foods. They should be taken alone because they decompose rapidly. Do not eat over-starchy food as a meal because it may lead to fermentation and poisoning of the body.

- Do not eat fats with proteins; avoid fatty meat; use learn meat, white meat, while meat like chicken, turkey, rabbits etc. and fish.

- Do not eat snacks between products regularly.

- Do not drink caffeinated products regularly.

- Do not take dessert like cake, custard at every meal.

- Avoid eating vegetable drenched with butter or cream,

- Eat fresh fruits and vegetables.

- Take honey, instead of sugar.

- Use cold pressed cooking oil like sunflower oil, cottonseed oil.

- Use vitamin and mineral supplements.

- Go for organically grown fruits and vegetables.

- Go for nuts like raw unsalted almonds, walnuts, cashew nuts, soya nuts.

- Always read labels and follow the manufacturer's guide when using any products.

Like we mentioned earlier, our habit practice could lead or poor health condition which may eventually hinder us from achieving our goal. We shall be examining few of the gradual devastating habits and practices of people.

1. Anxiety and worry: Many people tend to worry about so many things like where to live, how to pay their bills, what they would eat, how to be take care of their children, how to satisfy their husband or wife, and getting along with in laws, and how to get a better paid job or increasing in their career and many more. But they forget that worry and anxiety will not change the situation, rather it will increase tension and may eventually lead to hypertension.

2. The taking of hard drugs like cocaine, heroin, marijuana etc. could lead to serious mental problem and damage other functioning organs of the body system at old age.

3. Poor personal and environment hygiene: People who are unable to maintain a good personal and environment hygiene will expose themselves, their neighbors to numerous health hazards.

4. Nonchalant attitude to health related matters: Some people don't pay adequate attention to health related issues, ideas and discussion, they believe in natural health resuscitation thereby flout health rules and shun helpful ideas about their health.

5. Un-forgiveness and bitterness of mind: This is a negative attitude that many are known to be expert in; and it could cause both physical and spiritual illness like loss of appetite, loss of weight, peptic ulcer and psychosomatic problems.

6. Flirting and adultery: These immoral attitudes could lead to an individual contracting sexually transmitted diseases (STDS), HIV/ AIDS/ loss of self-respect and debasing of the dignity of manhood/womanhood.

7. Smoking of cigarettes, cigar, pipes and taking of snuff predisposes one to heart attacks and cancer, especially of the lugs.

8. Lack of exercise and laziness: These causes lots of psychological and physical setbacks because they increase one's chances of development diseases and increases the risk of obesity, diabetes and high blood pressure.

9. Self-pity and depression: These involved sadness, pessimism, preoccupation with personal problems and self-pity. It could also be accompanied be fatigue, excessive

sleeping, insomnia, anguish, crying and hopelessness, feeling of inadequacy or worthlessness, poor concentration or recurrent thoughts of death or suicide.

10. Anger: This triggers excessive production of certain hormones in the body which may result to stroke, heart attack, or paralysis. According to new research findings," all of the negative energy exerted in moments of anger isn't just a waste of time or a minor nuisance, it can lead to serious health complications that shorten lifespan and interfere with quality".

11. Lack of proper planning to balancing work and rest. This often leads to stress and confusion. Plan your work and avoid "biting more than you can chew". A day of getting enough rest is imperative to living a healthy lifestyle. When you do not release or get enough sleep you are putting yourself at the risk of illness as well as other dangerous side effects.

When you don't have through rest, concentrating, thinking, clearing and even remembering things becomes difficult. You may not notice this at first or blame it on your busy schedule; but the more sleep and rest you miss, the more serious these symptoms will become.

12. Bad feeding habits: overeating, eating at irregular times, skipping meals, eating the wrong types of food and unbalanced diet can predispose the person to exercise weight gain (obesity) and diabetes mellitus especially women. By their privileged position in preparing meals at home, women tend to eat in-between meals. This contributes greatly to their weight gain.

13. Fear of uncertainty: Many people have a lot of fears- fear of security, prevailing diseases in the community, failure in business, plan, work and careers, family breakup etc. What many do not know is that fear creates turmoil and chaos in our lives and contributes to ailment such as migraines. The human body is not meant to live in a state of fear. It is no wonder our health suffers.

CHAPTER FIVE

Some Possible Destructive Health Diseases Caused by These Habits.

High Blood Pressure O

Hypertension: This means high pressure or tension in the arteries. The arteries are the vessels that carry blood from the heart to all of tissues and organs of the body. Normal blood pressure is between 90/60 and below 140/90 m m h g. Thus, a blood pressure of 140/90mmhg and above is considered high. The top number which is known as the systolic blood pressure represents the pressure in the arteries as the heart contracts and pumps blood in to the arteries. Hypertension can lead to heart disease, stroke, paralysis and death predisposing factors include obesity, diabetes, emotional tension and stress.

Cancer

It is disease of all cells. It is an abnormal growth of the cells which tend to proliferate in an uncontrolled way. First, cells begin to grow out of control in the body. Second, those cells have the ability to travel from their original site to other location in the body. If the spread is not controlled, cancer can result to death, colon cancer, breast cancer (mostly woman) and prostate cancer (man).

Obesity

It is said to be the excessive accumulation of fat in the body which leads to great increase in weight. It is determined by the index of body man's index (BMI) where by weight in kilograms is divided by the height in meters squared. Overweight is defined as a BMI of 25 to 299, while obesity is defining as a BMI of 30 or more. The primary cause of obesity is consumption of more calories (food) than the body needs is uses. It is also caused by insufficient exercise. Obesity favors the development of many other diseases such as diabetes mellitus, gallstone, and hypertension, inguinal and hiatus hernia, varicose vein, uterine prolapsed and tiredness from overwork on the heart and lungs.

Tuberculosis.

Tuberculosis is a chronic bacterial infection. It is spread through the air and usually infects the lungs, although other organs and parts of the body can also be effected. Most people who are infected with tuberculosis at the latent stage harbor the bacterial without series of symptoms. Symptoms associate with this stage include weight loos, fever, night sweats and loss of appetite. It the affected individual is adequately treated, he gets cured. However, if left untreated, the latent TB will digenetic into the TB disease which has chronic and debilitating symptoms including severe cough, chest pain and body sputum.

Hiv/Aids

This is a chronic life threatening state or condition caused by the Human Immunodeficiency Virus (HIV). By damaging or destroying the cells of your immune system, HIV interferes with your body's ability to effectively fight off viral, bacterial and fungi that cause disease. This makes you more susceptible to certain types of cancer and to opportunistic infections. The term Acquired Immunodeficiency Syndrome (AIDS) is used to mean the latter stage of infected sharp instruments like needles, tattooing instrument, razor blade, shaving instrument and transfusion of infected blood could cause HIV/AIDS

Diabetes Mellitus

It is a metabolic disease characterized by exercise urination (with sugar in the urine), weight loos (due to excessive urination), excessive craving for water to and general body weakness. It has an attendant raise blood sugar level as a result of inadequate secretion of hormone called insulin. Contribution, factors as overeating, alcohol consumption, excessive craving for sweetened/sugary foods and drinks. This, if not well controlled will affects many other systems of the body and can cause diseases and /or untimely death. Change of feeding habits, regular exercise and weight shedding will go a long way to prevent this disease called diabetes.

CHAPTER SIX

The Remedies and Preventives Measures Against the Health Devastating Habits and Practices

1. We must learn to always carry our problems, cares and concerns to the Almighty God through prayers and trust in His mercy. Always obey every health rules.
2. Learn always to put a positive construction on every situation of life and on what people say to u or about you. This will help a great deal to keep your mind and heart healthy and sound; to think and act rightly always as well as develop the best attitude to life.
3. Rest: Sleeping 6 8hours a day is ideal.
4. Learn to always forgive every offence and make up your mind to do so
5. Go for routine checkup at six month intervals.
6. Do regular BP checkup at every available opportunity?
7. Eat good and balance diet with fruits and vegetables at regular intervals and at the right time.
8. Report any abnormal swelling or growth in any part of the body to doctor so as to prevent further damages to the body.
9. Always renew and strengthen your spirit by daily reading and meditating on God's Word. Remember that your body needs a healthy mind to function affection.

Body Exercise and Fitness

"For bodily exercise profit Is profitable unto all things, having promise of the life that now is and of which is to come." - 1 timothy 4:8

Exercise is an indispensable factor in any person's effort to maintain a healthy lifestyle.

Many people think or have misconception on the concept of exercise. They think exercise has to be vigorous to be beneficial but experts have said exercise done in a moderate form is actually more exercise comes in many forms from running to more cycling. Depending on factors such as your age, state of health and fitness goals, you could choose which form of exercise to engage in.

The followings are considered the possible benefits of bodily exercise.

1. Exercise helps people to maintain a healthy weighty by helping a person to burn excess calories and help prevent them from being stored as fat.
2. It helps people build stronger muscles. While most people begin losing muscle strength as early as age 25 to 30, it has been established that strength training can slow down or even reverse this process.
3. It also helps to lower the risk of illness such as heart disease, cancer, high blood pressures and diabetes.
4. It helps to increase bone strength and density. As this could also protect a woman from osteoporosis (a timing of the bones that often occurs during menopause). Women who strengthen their bones at a younger age are less likely to suffer from osteoporosis later in like.
5. Exercise improves emotional health; studies show that regular exercise can help people feel happier, less anxious and more related.

Cautions

Every though it is said and widely accept that the "combination of good nutrition and rest, moderate exercise is an indispensable factor in any person's effort to maintain a healthy lifestyle", we must understand that as important as exercise may be to our health, it can be counter-productive if done at the wrong way and at the wrong time. Now, after exercise if the following signs are observed then it means something is wrong somewhere: dizziness, headache, fainting attack, chronic fatigue, gasping for breath, excessive palpation, sleeplessness etc. This could simply mean that you're engaging in the wrong kind of exercise at the wrong time or in the wrong way. To avoid the risks associated with problematic exercise, the following guideline will the of help:

1. Choosing the most appropriate type for yourself. Understand your personal limitation and exercise accordingly. Note that you're not competing with anyone for a price.
2. Don't exercise when you're ill or feverish.
3. Don't engage in vigorous activities immediately after eating.
4. Adjust exercises to weather; be carefully especially of hot weather.
5. Aerobic exercise should always be started with proper warm up before the main exercise.
6. Wear proper clothing and shoes fit for exercise

Fitness

You are fit when there is a combination of qualities that enable you to perform vigorous physical and /or mental activities. While some think fitness means to be thin or lean. These are all wrong or myopic misconceptions.

Physical fitness

It is the capacity to cope with daily routines which include occupation and lifestyle routines without undue tiredness and with ample reserve of energy and zeal for recreation and emergencies. It also means when the body's capacity to carry out work and protect itself against disease, infection and the effects of physical discomforts like heat, cold and stress.

The followings are the components of physical fitness for the average person in moderately tasking occupation or lifestyle.

Flexibility

It is the ability it moves joints and stretch muscles through their full range of motion. A person who is very flexible for instance can bend over and touch the floor easily. Good flexibility in the joints can help prevent injuries through all stages of like. While is natural to lose some level of flexibility as we grow older, there are steps you can take to improve your flexibility through the years, for instance you can make up your mind to always stretch before and after every physical activity, stretching increases the range of motion and helps to stimulate muscle growth.

Muscle strength

It is the ability of muscle or group of muscle to act maximum force for brief time. It is the ability to perform some work maximum intensity at once e.g. lifting a heavy object.

Muscle Enhancement

It is the ability of a muscle to sustain a contraction or make multiple contractions over an extended period without undue fatigue. Put simple, it is the amount of time that your muscles are able to do a certain activity before they get tired.

Body Composition

It is the makeup of the body in terms of lean mass (muscle, bone, vita tissue and organs) and is an indication of one's level of health and fitness.

Cardio Respiratory Endurance

It is the ability of the heart and lungs to supply sufficient oxygen and nutrients to all areas of the body during sustained physical activity, aerobic endurance, and vascular endurance.

Medication Mistakes

You need to be well informed about the causes, consequence and cure for medication mistakes. Need to say that out of the millions of lives that are lost yearly, many are as a result of medication errors. More are admitted to emergency wards and Inversion Care Units on daily basis with diverse complications arising from medication mistake. It is so alarming that we must do everything possible to prevent its occurrence to us, our family and the society we live.

Medication is said to be a licensed drug taken to care or reduce symptoms of an illness or medical condition as well as the administration of such drug. Medication mistakes therefore refer to error that arise from the prescription and use of drugs.

The National Coordinating Council for Medication Error and Prevention (NCCMEP) in a more comprehensive and authoritative perspective defines medication mistake as "any preventable event that may cause or lead to inappropriate medication use or patient harm, while the medication is in the control of the health care professional, patient or consumer".

CHAPTER SEVEN

Various forms of medication mistake.

Mistake from Medical Practitioners

Mistakes with medication can occur from medical practitioners due to oversight or outright incompetence. Some too called doctors, nurses, pharmacists, chemists and specialists are not qualified; thus exhibit gross incompetence in their prescription. These quacks are only interested in making money by taking advantage of people's poverty, ignorance, gullibility and illiteracy. On the other hand, qualified medical practitioners who sometimes prescribe dispense and administer drugs carelessly. This often leads to serious errors.

Some mediation mistakes common with medical practitioners include incorrect drug selection for patient; wrong or confused drug names (this occurs primarily when two or more drug have similar appearance or similar name), Wrong dosage form or abbreviation, incorrect dosage calculations, incorrect dosage frequency, poorly written prescriptions; use of verbal orders (which are soon forgotten by patients); wrong medication combinations; administration of fake or expired drugs, dispensing without seeing a written order; failure to check the patient's identity prior to administration etc.

Mistakes from Patients/Drug Users.

This is the second medication mistake we will consider in our discussion because it is very common among people all over the world and this medication error with consumers include drug abuse, addiction and self-medication.

Drug Abuse and Addiction: Drug abuse is the use of illicit drugs or of prescription drugs (drugs prescribed by doctors) or over-the-counter drugs (drugs brought from chemists) for purposes other than those for which they are indicted or in a manner or in quantities other than directed.

Drug abuse is closely related to drug addiction, which is characterized by compulsive drug craving; seeking and use that persists even in that face of negative consequences. Many drug users are imperceptibly guilty of this. Because of the availability and usefulness of some drugs many people take them indiscriminately, paving the way for serious health problems.

Some drugs often abused include caffeine (a slightly bitter stimulant found in coffee tea, kola nut, ilex plants and in small amounts in cocoa), Analgesics /Antipyretics (pain relieving and fever reducing drugs such as aspirin, Paracetamol, Acetaminophen, Opium, Morphine, Heroin and Codeine), Antibiotics (these include drugs such as Amplicon, Ampicillin and Tetracycline), Nicotine (a stimulant found predominantly tobacco and in lower quantities in tomatoes, eggplant and green pepper) inhalers (especially for Asthma patients), Sedatives/ Tranquilizers/ Depressants (drugs used to relieve anxiety, restlessness, sleeplessness etc.) and Steroids (drugs administered in small quantities by physicians to treat conditions that occurs when the body produces abnormally low amount of testosterone, but often abused especially by athletes for muscle building and performance enhancement).

The abuse and misuse of these otherwise useful drugs can lead to serious health problems such as dehydration, insomnia, restlessness, tumors, convulsions, amnesia, high blood pressure, paralysis, cancer, brain damage or even death.

Self-Medication: It is self-prescription, dispensing and administration of drugs without a medical expert's direction or supervision. This is tantamount to playing the role of your own doctor. Most drugs users assume that with a few physical signs and symptoms, they can easily diagnose and ascertain their type of illness and the medication to take for the curs. This can be very dangerous and in fact deadly.

As much as possible, self-medication should be avoided for the following reasons:

1. Illness sometimes has deeper roots than what we see physically and if you don't see a competent doctor or pharmacist as soon as possible, the illness may degenerate to fatal state.

2. Some illnesses have similar symptoms.

3. Self-medication could lead to dangerous drug interactions. A. drug interactions occurs when two or more medicines combine in your body in a way that is potentially harmful or dangerous. Since you're not a medical expert, you may not have knowledge of drugs that shouldn't interact with one another. Self-prescription and administration could therefore pose serious health risks.

4. Some drug, are food sensitive" and this often leads to dangerous drugs food interaction. This happens when the food you eat affects the ingredients in a medicine. This is why some medicines are required to be taken on an empty stomach (1 hour before eating o N 2 hour after eating). Only a competent professional can tell you which is which

5. Human body systems do not always function some way. It is risky to assume that a drug will be good for you simply because it was effective for someone who had similar illness. You might be allergic to some drugs which work for someone else.

6. Medication Mistakes with Patients /Drug Users Not Completing the Dosage a Prescribed Medicine.

    This is also a very common mistake among drugs users. Often because a sickness appears to have been healed while medicines still being taken, drugs users tend to discard the remaining dosage with the belief that it's no longer necessary to continues with the medicine.

7. The Mistake of Patronizing Unapproved but Cheap Drug stores, Pharmacies and Hospitals.

8. The Mistake of Leaving the Doctor's Office without Enough Information on Prescription and Drugs.

9. The Mistake of Not Storing Drugs as Directed.

10. The Mistake of Not Taking Drugs at the Right Time or in the Right Quantity.

11. Keeping Different Tablet in the Same Jar.

12. Mixing Food-Sensitive Drugs with Food.

13. Using Multiple Pharmacies, they can't screen for drug interaction because they won't have a complete list of all the medication you are on", a doctor explained.

Preventing Medication Mistake /Errors

Michael Cohen, a medical expert says "you should expect to count on the health system to keep you safe, but there are also steps you can take to look after yourself and family". Even though medication errors are common, yet they are preventable."

Herein are some of these steps, as suggested by professional health counsellors:

1. Always ask for written instruction to take with you. Don't just leave the doctor's office with verbal instructions? Ask him to write because you may forget or confuse part of the verbal instructions.

2. Inspect your medication when you receive them from the pharmacy. Check them out. Look at the appearance- cooler, shape, markings; smell it. Does it look or smell differently? Are the directions on the bottle different from what the doctor told you in the office?

3. Check the medicine name. Many drugs sound alike and are spelt similarly. Be sure to double-check that the medication prescription is what you picked up from the pharmacy.

4. Save package inserts/wrapping: Don't throw away the package insert or outer wrapper that held your medication. You may need it for dosing instructions and for information about contraindication (what drugs should not be used in conjunction with the medicine).

5. Question price changes: If the cost of your medication was different from the last time you purchased it, question it! You may find that it is the wrong medication.

6. Inform your doctor about other medications. Tell your doctor about all the medications you are taking; prescription and over-the-counter, including nutritional supplements. If you do not tell your doctor about all the medications you are taking, you may be risking a bad drug interaction.

7. Ask if there are interactions with any other medicines or dietary supplement (including vitamins or beverages or food).

8. Make a list of your medicine before leaving the hospital. Go over your list of medications with your doctor, including dosing information. Make a list and take any notes that will help check the list or write the list for you.

9. Tell your doctor about medication allergies.

10. Handle sample medications carefully: Sample do not come with instructions on the packaging or other important information you may need. If you doctor gives you samples, he will typically write the instructions for you. Place those instructions in the package; if possible wrap them around the package with a rubber band.

11. Check medication expiration dates: Throw away any medication that has expired.

12. As much as possible, keep medicines in their original labelled containers.

13. Never combine different medicine in some bottle.

14. Do not patronize quack doctors or pharmacists.

15. As much as possible, do not resort to self-medication.

16. Never take medication which was prescribed for another person.

17. Do not store medication in direct light, heat or humidity.

18. Ensure to take at least a full glass of water when taking tablets to avoid dehydration.

19. Don't chew, crush, break or mix tablets or capsules unless your doctor has told you to do so. Some medicines have a special coating and will not work properly unless they are swallowed whole.

20. Carefully read and follow the directions on the label and the directions from your doctor, pharmacist or other health care professional. If your doctor specifies taking your medicine before, with or after food, it is important you follow these instructions.

21. Measure your medicine carefully (e.g. use a medicine spoon or take only the recommended number of puffs). If is important to tale only recommended dose of your medicines as too much can be harmful and too little might prevent the medicine from working properly. For liquid medicines, remember to shake the bottle before measuring out the correct amount, as some liquid medicines may settle at the base of the bottle.

22. Do not take medication in the dark where you can easily pick up the wrong container.

23. Always pray in faith to God Almighty before or after taken your medication because medications take care of our health problems, it is God Almighty that heals.

CONCLUSION

The qualities of a good home are a clean and lovely environment. A clean environment makes for good health. Besides, nerves cannot be smoothed in a dirty and chaotic environment; neither can rest be had in such a place. For the purpose of your safety and proper health condition, you must make sure you take adequate care of your environment. This is because many of the result of dirty home and poor environment conditions. This is one great challenge that must be tackled individually and collectively if we want to have a healthy and happy home. Remember it is said," there is no place like home". This is true only if the environment is properly taken care of.

Care of Our Environment and Home

1. Sweep the surrounding everyday keep paths clean.
2. Empty all refuse from the house and its surrounding. This should be alone daily.
3. Keep the refuse bin clean and ensure that refuse is dumped into the bin and covered properly.
4. Do not leave empty cans, broken plates, cups, bottles, wastes and food stuff lying about in the surroundings.
5. Clean the drainage properly and do not allow stagnant water in your home/ environment.
6. Sweep and clean the floor regularly; remove all debris including bits of sponge, broom or soap from the bathroom daily.
7. Take towels out in the sun after use. Do not keep wet towel in your living room; it gives a bad smell to the room.
8. Open the window to allow air in and out of the bedroom.
9. Wash the bathtub and wash hand basin daily after use.
10. To transform your home, make effort to acquire useful ideas on home keeping. Read books and magazine on home making since home differ; your plan will depend on the kind of home you live.

www.ingramcontent.com/pod-product-compliance
Lightning Source LLC
Chambersburg PA
CBHW060900260726
48661CB00008B/3362